ASPERGERS SYNDROME

The Easy-to-understand and Practical Guide for Parents

(Making Way for Asperger's Syndrome)

Debbra Prince

Published by Tomas Edwards

© **Debbra Prince**

All Rights Reserved

Aspergers Syndrome: The Easy-to-understand and Practical Guide for Parents (Making Way for Asperger's Syndrome)

ISBN 978-1-990268-73-1

All rights reserved. No part of this guide may be reproduced in any form without permission in writing from the publisher except in the case of brief quotations embodied in critical articles or reviews.

Legal & Disclaimer

The information contained in this book is not designed to replace or take the place of any form of medicine or professional medical advice. The information in this book has been provided for educational and entertainment purposes only.

The information contained in this book has been compiled from sources deemed reliable, and it is accurate to the best of the Author's knowledge; however, the Author cannot guarantee its accuracy and validity and cannot be held liable for any errors or omissions. Changes are periodically made to this book. You must consult your doctor or get professional medical advice before using any of the suggested remedies, techniques, or information in this book.

Upon using the information contained in this book, you agree to hold harmless the Author from and against any damages, costs, and expenses, including any legal fees potentially resulting from the application of any of the information provided by this guide. This disclaimer applies to any damages or injury caused by the use and application, whether directly or indirectly, of any advice or information presented, whether for breach of contract, tort, negligence, personal injury, criminal intent, or under any other cause of action.

You agree to accept all risks of using the information presented inside this book. You need to consult a professional medical practitioner in order to ensure you are both able and healthy enough to participate in this program.

Table of Contents

INTRODUCTION 1

CHAPTER 1: SYMPTOMS 4

CHAPTER 2: THE DIAGNOSIS... 17

CHAPTER 3: ASPERGERS SYNDROME BEHAVIORAL ASPECT 52

CHAPTER 4: CAUSES ASPERGER'S SYNDROME 79

CHAPTER 5: TREATMENT OPTIONS AND INTERVENTIONS 88

CHAPTER 6: FACTS AND MYTHS ABOUT ASPERGER'S SYNDROME 100

CHAPTER 7: AFFECTING THE COMMUNICATION OF A PERSON WITH AS 108

CHAPTER 8: THE FUTURE IS BRIGHT............................... 117

CHAPTER 9: EFFECTS OF THE SYNDROME ON SPEECH AND LANGUAGE 123

CONCLUSION 143

Introduction

In this book, I am going to describe some common facts about Asperger syndrome. In my first section, I tried to explain what Asperger syndrome really is and how it is different from other kinds of neurological disorder. Asperger syndrome has many symptoms that come into existence only when a child approaches his or her middle or high school. It really becomes mandatory to recognize the early signs of this syndrome so that the child should be provided proper cure and treatment and that's why I have explained some common symptoms of this syndrome. Many parents are not even sure whether their child is suffering from Asperger syndrome or other kind of neurological disorder. This book can really help them to understand what really Asperger syndrome is and how to identify it through analysing some of the common symptoms.

Next, I have written about the common cause of this disease so that you should understand it well. In my next section "Impact of Asperger syndrome on Children's normal life" I have give a thorough explanation about the various challenges an Asperger child has to face in his life like social challenges, communication challenges, cognition challenges, sensory and motor challenges. I also explained about the social, communication, and cognition issues that an Asperger child has.

Then, in my next section called "Treatments for Asperger syndrome" I have described about some of the common treatment and prevention techniques that should be adopted in case of Asperger syndrome for giving your child a chance to grow and socialize normally. I have described about the various techniques of treatment like Applied Behaviour Analysis, Verbal Behaviour Therapy, Pivotal Response Treatment, Cognitive Behaviour Therapy,

Occupational Therapy, and finally Physical Therapy.

You should have attained a good knowledge at this point of reading my book, so I have provided some basic tips to the parents to give their child a chance to live and grow. Finally, I have tried to provide a motivating conclusion to my book so that you, as a parent of Asperger child, should not only become alert about how to treat your child but can also adopt the techniques of my book for his or her goodwill.

Chapter 1: Symptoms

The symptoms of Asperger's disorder vary, and may range from mild to severe disorders as a child grows.
Symptoms during childhood:
Asperger's Syndrome is often first noticed by parents when the child starts preschool and starts interacting with other kids. Asperger's kids may:
Not like changes
Lack empathy
Lack inborn social skills
Not be able to distinguish tone pitch and accent of speech
Not understand sarcasm or jokes
Have a flat tone when speaking
Have a formal speaking style like using more complex words
Talk too much about their favorite topic while having one-sided conversations
Avoid eye contact
Have facial expressions that are not usual

Be interested in only a few things and not others

Be more sensitive to or over-influenced by noise, light, or textures

Teen years:

Many of the above symptoms continue through teenage years. Communication skills remain poor, and although they may start to learn social skills, they have trouble reading other's behaviors.

Kids with Asperger's will want to have friends, but may feel timid about approaching others. They may feel different from others. Where other teens pose to be cool, kids with Asperger's find this depressing, and they are drained emotionally to fit within. They may act immature and trust everyone easily, which can cause them to be exploited. They often withdraw themselves from society, but this isolation can cause depression and anxiety.

Some children with Asperger's Syndrome are capable of making a few close friends in school. They are not interested in following others who can be helpful in making them leaders, not the followers, in the classroom.

Adulthood:

Asperger's Syndrome stays with a person throughout their life. With the passage of time, it becomes stable, and the situation improves. As adults are more capable of understanding their weaknesses and strengths, they can improve their social skills.

Few traits that are typical of children with Asperger Syndrome, such as awareness to detail and focused interests, improve chances of a successful career. Numerous people with Asperger's are enthralled with technology, and a common career choice is engineering. But scientific careers are by no means the only areas where people with Asperger's excel. Indeed, many respected historical figures have been reported to display Asperger's-like traits, including Wolfgang Amadeus Mozart, Albert Einstein, Marie Curie, and Thomas Jefferson.

General problems:

Social skills problem: Children with Asperger's typically have trouble interacting with others, and they behave awkwardly while dealing with people. They find it difficult to start and continue a conversation, so they cannot make friends easily.

Repetitive behaviors: Children that have Asperger's Syndrome may develop odd, recurring motions, such as snapping or twisting their finger.

Unusual preoccupations or rituals: A child with this syndrome may become set in their rituals and be resistant to changing them, as in dressing in a particular order.

Difficulties in Communication: It is common that people with Asperger's Syndrome are unable to make eye contact while they are speaking to someone. For them, it might be difficult to use facial expressions or gestures, and to understand someone's body language. They may also have difficulty understanding the context of the language and the use of language in its literal meaning.

Limited range of interests: Children with Asperger's Syndrome may develop a strong or even obsessive interest in limited areas, such as specific sports, news, or collecting objects.

Coordination problems: They may have awkward movements.

Skilled or Talented Children: Many children with Asperger's Syndrome are extremely talented or skilled in a specific area, such as geography or music.

Genetic Causes:

The precise cause of Asperger's Syndrome is not yet known. However, it is presumed to be inherited, since it runs in the families. It is not clear whether a particular gene variation plays any role in Asperger's Syndrome, or multiple variations in genes plus environmental factors combine to influence the development of this complex condition.

It is a disorder in which brain development plays a role. Researchers have noticed certain differences in the structure and function of particular regions of the brain. These differences arise during the development of the brain in the fetus, when there is migration of brain cells into their proper places.

THEORY OF MIND: This is the ability to understand the unique ideas, emotions, and perceptions of other people, and to react to them. The mirror neuron system which is involved in this process is normally active both when a particular action is performed, and when others are observed performing the same actions. This mirror neuron system is impaired in individuals with Asperger's.

Frequency:

It is only recently that Asperger's Syndrome has begun to be recognized as a unique disorder. The exact number of affected people is still unknown. Asperger's Syndrome is more general then autism, so it is estimated that anywhere from one in 250 to one in 10,000 children have Asperger's Syndrome in the US and Canada alone. Males are more likely to be affected than females, and the age in which it is usually diagnosed in children is between 2 to 6.

Diagnosis:

If some or all of the symptoms are present in a child then doctors perform a complete medical and neurological exam to start an evaluation process. Many individuals who have Asperger's show low muscle tone and dyspraxia, or issues with coordination. The doctor may use a number of tests, such as x-rays and blood tests, as there is no specific test for Asperger's Syndrome. These tests will determine whether there is any physical disorder that is causing the symptoms to occur. If no physical cause is found, the child is referred to a child specialist, or sometimes a child and adolescent psychiatrist or psychologist, pediatric neurologist, developmental-behavioral pediatrician, or some other health specialist who can specifically diagnose and start treatment of Asperger's Syndrome. The diagnosis of the doctor is based on the developmental level of the child, their speech and behavior, and their capability to socialize with people around them. Parents, teachers, and other adults familiar with the child also play a major part in directing the doctor toward treatment, as they all are familiar with the child's behavior.

Your primary care provider may refer your child to a specialist for testing that includes:

Psychological assessment. This covers intellectual functioning and learning style. The more common tests include the intelligence quotient or IQ Test, motor skill tests, and personality assessment tests.

Communication assessment. This includes the evaluation of speech and formal language, with the purpose of finding out how normal the child's understanding and language are, and how they communicate their ideas. Nonverbal forms of communication and nonliteral skills are also tested, such as comprehension of metaphor or humor. Volume, stress, and pitch of the child's speech are also measured and compared to normative standards.

Psychiatric examination. The family of a child with Asperger's Syndrome is also interviewed by the doctor, as well as peer relationships, their reactions to new situations, and their understanding of the feelings of others. Indirect communication that includes teasing and satire is tested too. In psychiatric examinations, the doctor may observe the behavior of the child at home and in school. The conditions of anxiety and depression that are more commonly found in Asperger's Syndrome patients are also evaluated.

Treatments for Asperger's:

Medication: There is no specific medication for Asperger's, and in fact most people with Asperger's Syndrome are not on medication. In a few cases, to treat specified symptoms such as anxiety, depression, hyperactivity, and obsessive-compulsive disorder, specific drugs are used. Stimulants for inattention and hyperactivity may be prescribed to some Asperger's patients. For persevering obsessions, SSRIs such as Paxil, Prozac, or Zoloft may help. Depression and anxiety, often associated with Asperger's, can also be treated with SSRIs. In children with stereotyped actions, disturbance, and distinctive thinking, a low dose of an antipsychotic such as Risperidone may be prescribed.

Psychotherapy: Therapists who try hard to make intense emotional contact at early stages may provide disappointing results, so therapy should start slowly and keep to whatever emotional intensity the patient can handle. Playing is also helpful, if the therapist correctly uses it to teach interaction. It can also be used by the therapist as a break from tense emotions. Group therapy is also very helpful for both kids and adults. Support groups may also help, as a place to share experiences with people who may have gone through something similar.

Special Education: The child is educated in such a way so as to meet their unique educational needs. As Asperger's covers a broad range of ability levels, the school should ideally individualize programming for each child with Asperger's. Educators must be made aware that the student may mumble or avoid eye contact, and the child should be informed well in advance about any changes that will take place in the school routine. The student may continue on through college or even further. Kids with Asperger's usually have raw and unskilled social behavior, so they may not behave well in a class with emotional disturbances like aggression. Some children do very well with other students who have developmental disorders, while some may excel in routine classes along with normal students, though some extra support will always be needed. This may include an instructional assistant, resource room, or extra training for the primary teacher.

Social Skills Therapies: Social skill therapies are done by a psychologist, counselor, speech pathologist, or social worker. These therapies are helpful in building social skills and the ability to read verbal and non-verbal cues that are so often lacking in those with Asperger's. This is a very important part of treatment at all ages, since a child must learn body language just like an adult learning a foreign language. They have to be taught rules for eye contact, socially appropriate personal space, and slang. Cultivating a global understanding is difficult, but they can still be taught to look for particular signs that point towards the emotional state of other individuals. Social skills should ideally be taught in small group settings.

Modification in Behavior: Supporting positive behavior and diminishing the behaviors that causes problems is a major step in treating Asperger's Syndrome. Speech, physical, or occupational therapy are also used to increase the child's functional abilities, and these therapies are specially designed to get results.

Outlook for People with Asperger's Syndrome:

Children with Asperger's are at risk for developing other conditions, such as depression, ADHD, and schizophrenia. A number of treatment options are available to cure these conditions. As they have average or more than average intelligence level, most of the people with this syndrome can work very well. They may have a problem to socialize throughout adulthood.

Prevention:

Asperger's Syndrome runs in families through genetics, so it can neither be prevented nor cured. However, if diagnosed in its early stages, the function and quality of life of the individual can be improved with various therapies and treatments.

Chapter 2: The Diagnosis

Getting an Official Asperger's Syndrome Diagnosis

Here we will discuss the issues and techniques surrounding diagnosis of Asperger's Syndrome. The issue has become a bit of a minefield with many doctors and general practitioners refusing to allow people the opportunity of an official diagnosis.

Many people have already taken the free online AQ Test, which gives people the opportunity to get an initial insight into the degree of their autistic traits without the hassle or expense of going for a medical consultation. While it gives a good general indication as to where one is on the Autism Spectrum, it is not a substitute for an official diagnosis.

We have written this post to try and represent diagnosis perspectives from a UK and US angle; however, we are aware that the advice we give may be applicable to all countries (and states).

The landscape of diagnosis is continually changing with new legislation, changes to insurance policies etc. Some people in the US have been able to get a diagnosis with their existing insurance whilst others have not. Often people end up paying to have a diagnosis. Because things differ so much, you will need to do your own research in your place of living to determine the best course of action.

Why get an official diagnosis?

The question of whether one needs to get an official diagnosis needs to be carefully considered.

For many, it is not necessary to go through the trauma of trying to get an official diagnosis. Taking online tests, reading about symptoms and understanding the intricacies of the condition can be enough. Please bear in mind that if you choose to go down the path of official diagnosis, you may not get a correct diagnosis. Sometimes people can get misdiagnosed (for example, with mental health problems such as schizophrenia). Often, doctors identify the most prominent symptom and give a diagnosis based on that alone. For example, the impaired motor skills aspect of Asperger's is often diagnosed as dyspraxia without taking into account other symptoms that may exist alongside it.

Before the changes to the Diagnostic Statistic Manual (which we will discuss later) it was easier for people with Asperger's to get support. However, now that Asperger's is grouped together with classic Autism, there is less support for people with Asperger's. While this still differs from country (and state to state), it is important to do your own research. You will find there is more specific information about details of services in the UK and US when you begin to do your own research.

The kind of support you may be able to get is:

Social Security Income

Disability Allowance

Community Care.

People with Asperger's are also entitled to disability rights, where they can request specific accommodations in their workplace.

How to get officially diagnosed with Asperger's

The first step in getting an official diagnosis is speaking with your GP (doctor). They have the capacity to make referrals to either a:

Neuropsychologist

Psychologist

Psychiatrist or

Social Worker.

Very often it is the case that GP's are not so familiar with Asperger's Syndrome, so it is important to do a bit of research before you turn up for your appointment. The National Autism Society have done a great job of putting together this information pack for GP's: www.autism.org.uk/~/media/NAS/Documents/Working-with/Health/GPs-guide-to-adults-with-Asperger-syndrome.ashx. It may be worth your printing this out and bringing it with you to your appointment.

Due to insurance issues or budget restrictions within the health system, it is possible that your GP may not be able to refer you — in which case you could try to connect directly with a specialist.

In the US, you can find state by state information here: http://grasp.org/page/statebystate-help.

Or if you live in the UK you can check out the British Psychological Society for a list of Psychiatrists or Neuropsychologists: http://www.bps.org.uk/psychology-public/find-psychologist/find-psychologist.

In both of these cases it is advisable to seek out someone that is familiar with, or specialises in, Asperger's Syndrome.

Please bear in mind that the way assessments are carried out are not standard. You can find more guidelines that professionals should be following at: http://www.nice.org.uk/guidance/CG142.

There are also occasional opportunities at universities and other research institutions that may be available. These are often performed for free but you would need to do your own investigation to see what is possible in your area.

Do your research

I live my life on the premise that I am responsible for it, not my parents, not the medical establishment and not the government. Given that there are disturbingly high rates of misdiagnosis in the medical system, it is important to forearmed, so you can challenge things if you feel you are being misinformed.

According to this article http://www.cbsnews.com/news/12-million-americans-misdiagnosed-each-year-study-says/ 12 million Americans are misdiagnosed every year. This amounts to 1 in 20 adult patients, and in half of the misdiagnosis cases there is the potential for severe harm.

So do your research, search the internet and go prepared for any engagement with the medical system.

Free Online Testing Resources

AQ Test

One of the most common ways people get diagnosed for Asperger's Syndrome or High-functioning Autism is by using the Autism Quotient or AQ Test.

The test was published by Simon Baron-Cohen and his colleagues at the Autism Research Centre in Cambridge, UK, in 2001.[1] The test takes into account all of the factors listed above and aims "to investigate whether adults of average intelligence have symptoms of autism or one of the other autism spectrum conditions".[2] Although not intended to be a diagnostic test,[3] it has become very popular as a tool for preliminary self-diagnosis of Asperger's,[4] and further papers have indicated that it could be used clinically to screen test for the condition (suggesting that a diagnosis of Asperger's can be ruled out for those scoring less than 26).[2]

The test itself consists of questions in a 'forced choice' format, meaning that the answer is ultimately an 'agree' or 'disagree' with a given statement. It covers the five main areas associated with the Autism Spectrum: social skills; communication skills; imagination; attention to detail; and attention switching/tolerance of change.[5] Possibly due to the popularity of the test for preliminary self-diagnosis, versions of the AQ for children[6] and adolescents[7] have also been published.

The test can be taken by anyone for free at www.AspergersTestSite.com.

We've also developed a version of the AQ Test which can be used on mobile devices; there are versions for iPhone, iPad and Android.

[1] Woodbury-Smith M.R., Robinson J., Wheelwright S., Baron-Cohen S. (2005). "Screening adults for Asperger Syndrome using the AQ: a preliminary study of its diagnostic validity in clinical practice" (PDF). J. Autism Dev. Disord. **35**(3):331–335. doi:10.1007/s10803-005-3300-7. PMID 16119474. Retrieved 20/10/2010.

[2] Woodbury-Smith M.R., Robinson J., Wheelwright S., Baron-Cohen S. (2005). "Screening adults for Asperger Syndrome using the AQ: a preliminary study of its diagnostic validity in clinical practice" (PDF). J. Autism Dev. Disord. **35**(3):331–335. doi:10.1007/s10803-005-3300-7. PMID 16119474. Retrieved 21/10/2011.

[3] Take the AQ Test, Embarrassing Bodies website, Channel 4, 2011. Accessed 21/10/2011.

[4] Autism Spectrum Quotient at Answers About Autism website (part of Better Your Health), 2006.

[5] Hoekstra R.A., Bartels M., Cath D.C., Boomsma D.I. (2008). "Factor structure, reliability and criterion validity of the Autism-Spectrum Quotient (AQ): a study in Dutch population and patient groups". J. Autism Dev. Disord. **38**(8):1555–1566. doi:10.1007/s10803-008-0538-x.

PMC 2516538. PMID 18302013.

[6] Auyeung B., Baron-Cohen S., Wheelwright S., Allison C. (2008). "The Autism Spectrum Quotient: Children's Version (AQ-Child)" (PDF). J. Autism Dev. Disord. **38**(7):1230–1240. doi:10.1007/s10803-007-0504-z.

PMID 18064550. Retrieved 21/10/2011.

[7] Baron-Cohen S., Hoekstra R.A., Knickmeyer R., Wheelwright S. (2006). "The Autism-Spectrum Quotient (AQ)— adolescent version" (PDF). J. Autism Dev.

Disord. **36**(3):343–350. doi:10.1007/s10803-006-0073-6.

Other Online Tests

The nice thing about online tests is that you can take this from the comfort of your own home.

Here is a list of other online tests, you may want to consider looking at:

Broad Autism Phenotype Test – According to the website "This questionnaire is designed to measure the mild autistic traits present in people who are not actually autistic but have a genetic predisposition to autism."

Aspie Quiz — A slight variation of the AQ Test; this will measure neurodiverse and neurotypical traits in adults.

Mind in the Eyes Test – This is a test that evaluates capacity to read facial expressions.

Telling someone that you think they may have Asperger's Syndrome

Firstly, I would like to say that it has been a difficult decision to sit down and write. "How do I tell some they may have Asperger's?" is a question that I get asked a lot on this site and it is always a difficult one to answer.

I usually try to avoid giving specific advice, because I don't know the individual involved. So rather than providing you with the 'correct' answer or the correct things to say, I will try and leave it open and cover the issue from several angles and then leave it open for debate. At the end of the day, I believe we all need to make informed decisions about this subject.

Before I go into this issue, I think it's important for us to look inside, about why it's important to tell the person they may have Asperger's. I have seen relationship situations where one partner uses the 'fact' that the other partner is on the spectrum to win arguments or just to be right and I believe this is totally the wrong motivation.

In many cases the actual diagnosis or awareness of whether a person has Asperger's Syndrome can be liberating. Understanding why one behaves and thinks the way one does can give the person a lot of self-acceptance. With that knowledge, an individual can also seek out techniques and therapies that can support them to have a better quality of life. Now this is a good motivation to make someone aware.

But……. it really depends on the individual. Some people are really not open to feedback. They do not invite it and they are really not open to it if it comes unsolicited. So if your loved one is in this bracket you need to be super aware because in trying to help, you run the danger of pushing the person away in the process and this is really not what you want. In these cases it can often be better to let the person come to their own conclusions and journey of self-discovery. However, if the person is more open and seeks advice, it can be easier.

I have talked to Renee Salas about this issue and we both agree it is a loaded but important subject. Renee has an excellent post where she discusses this issue from the point of view a parent. She suggests a number of questions one should ask oneself before going into the issue. I quite like them so I thought I would add them here. Try asking yourself these questions as part of the decision process about whether to talk to the person or not:

Do I think this person would want to know?

Do I think this person should know because it's what I want? Or is it what he/she would want?

Do I want to tell this person because I think it will make things easier for him/her? (E.g. are they lost and struggling in areas, confused at their inability to 'fit in' or succeed?)

What is this person's current view of Autism? This is a biggy. Autism still has so much negative stigma attached. If the person is not privy to the Autism community that we are a part of (i.e. bloggers/FB'ers/Twitterers who are working to bring the positives and successes to the forefront from an autistic point of view) their reaction would probably be one of anger. Then possibly fear and denial.

Am I looking at this person as an individual, taking into consideration: family, friends, social circles, job/career?

Is he/she overly concerned with what others think? Is he/she the type of person who might feel shame and worry over being stigmatised as a 'person with a disability'?

If the answers to the above convince you that it would be right to talk to the person or make them aware, here are a few ways I can think of to playfully or gently make him/her aware of the symptoms of Asperger's Syndrome.

Watch movies on Asperger's Syndrome and Autism

Many times people in the general public are not aware of the symptoms and mannerisms of Asperger's. By watching movies and TV series that portray the character and personality of people with the condition, you can initially raise awareness. Often the person will recognise traits in the characters and it may be a way to very slowly raise awareness to the point where the subject can eventually be broached.

Here is a list of Autism and Aspergers related movies: http://www.aspergerstestsite.com/598/aspergers-movies

Make the taking of a test a playful activity

So, just like any game, often people like to partake as a bit of fun. Taking turns to take the Test for Aspergers can be a playful way to get someone to take an initial screening assessment. You can also send the link to someone and say something like "I got a score of x, am curious what you got". The important thing is that it has to be done playfully and you have to feel the person is open to receive the information. It should also not be done in a competitive way that comes across as "I am normal and you have something wrong with you."

The test is available on our website as well as a Google Android or IOS application.

Highlighting the genius

To many there is a big stigma with having Asperger's; it is deemed as something negative. But if you would intentionally mention the positive aspects of people who have Asperger's and suggest that your friend has similar traits, it may be a way to get that person to open up to the possibility.

Read this — it sounds like you

Well, this isn't my idea, but I found it on a forum. Some became aware of their nature by someone emailing them a link that said, "Read this, it sounds like you." Apparently, this casual suggestion left the person free to decide for themselves. It also didn't cause offense or bring up defenses because the person could see why it sounded like them. You could try a similar thing, giving them a link to a good introduction to an article about Asperger's such as: http://www.autism.org.uk/about-autism/autism-and-asperger-syndrome-an-introduction/what-is-asperger-syndrome.aspx.

Talking directly to the person

Talking directly to the person is all about the right approach.

The National Autistic Society recommend that you consider who is the right person to broach the subject. For example, the person may be more able to accept the results of the conversation if it comes from a friend or sibling rather than a parent. The NAS encourage one to carefully plan out what will be said in a way that is diplomatic. You can check out this article, which has a few good ideas on how to handle the issue: http://www.autism.org.uk/about-autism/autism-and-asperger-syndrome-an-introduction/what-is-asperger-syndrome/asperger-syndrome-broaching-the-subject.aspx.

So, as I said at the beginning, this is a very difficult and sensitive issue to talk about. You will need to adopt any of the ideas to the person, but remember they are only ideas. Talking to people and communicating difficult issues is a fine art. No one can truly teach you this art; it's something you need to develop inside of yourself. If you are not confident that what you say or do will be well received, perhaps you should not. In such cases, just respect the fact that the person will be open to face or acknowledge things in themselves when they are ready.

Adults with Asperger's – Getting a late diagnosis

By Cynthia Kim

More and more adults are being diagnosed with Autism Spectrum Disorder (ASD) in their thirties, forties and beyond. Not surprisingly, one of the most common ways that adults realise they are on the spectrum is in the wake of having a child diagnosed with ASD.

Some parents start out researching Autism as an explanation for their child's struggles and realise that an ASD diagnosis would explain a lot about their own life, too. The first clue for others is when a professional who works with their child mentions that Autism can run in families. Regardless of how it happens, there is often a sense of disbelief at that initial Aha! moment.

I remember the exact moment I first thought I might have Asperger's Syndrome. I was listening to an NPR story about David Finch, the author of "The Journal of Best Practices". Finch described an online quiz that his wife asked him to take because she recognised so many Aspie traits in him.

As he and his wife described the quiz questions, for the first time I realised that Asperger's Syndrome (AS) is more than just social awkwardness and that I'm more than just painfully shy. The symptoms that stood out most for me were the ones I'd never known were 'symptoms' of anything other than my personality: attachment to routine, resistance to change, special interests, a need to be alone. I found myself nodding along with the program, shocked at how much I had in common with Finch, and yet not quite believing I could have gone four decades without realizing something so critical about myself.

The first thing I did was search for a screening quiz like the one described in the radio program. I took the AQ and the Aspie Quiz, certain that one of them would prove me wrong, even as I repeatedly scored in the high range for AS traits on each.

I sat there at my desk for long minutes. Could it be possible that I'd been autistic all my life and not known it? I'd always known that I was different. I'd been labelled 'shy', 'weird', 'introverted', 'geeky'. But what if I wasn't just weird? What if this thing called Asperger's Syndrome explained everything about me that was different?

That was an exciting thought. If it was true, it gave me a whole new way of thinking about my life. But the excitement soon wore off and I was faced with what to do with this realization. It turns out there aren't many resources for adults with ASD, especially those who aren't formally diagnosed.

Is a diagnosis necessary?

A diagnosis opens the door to services at school and home for children, but what about for adults? If you've made it into mid-life without a diagnosis, you may find yourself wondering if getting diagnosed really matters. I went back and forth for months on the question of whether to seek a professional diagnosis. Eventually I decided to pursue a diagnosis, primarily for peace of mind. I needed to know that I wasn't imagining everything.

There are many reasons you may choose to pursue a diagnosis as an adult: to access services, to request accommodations at work or school, or to increase the likelihood that therapy or counselling takes your ASD traits into account. Whatever your reason, it's important to be aware that the diagnostic process is more challenging for adults than for children.

Many adults run into difficulties with access. There are still few professionals qualified to diagnose adults. The process is often expensive and not covered by health insurance. Misdiagnosis is common. And some adults choose not to seek a formal diagnosis out of concern that it may lead to stigma or bias, or create practical limitations like not being able to join the military or having parental rights questioned.

The self-discovery process

Obviously, this is a decision that you'll want to give a lot of thought to. As you do, it can be helpful to spend time on self-discovery, testing out your suspicion that you're on the spectrum through research and introspection.

Self-discovery can include:

Learning more about ASD in adults: if you have a child with ASD, you're familiar with ASD traits. While the diagnostic criteria are the same for all ages, autism looks different in adults than it does in children. As we age, we develop a range of coping mechanisms that can mask typical symptoms, making them harder to identify. There can also be gender-related differences. Good sources of information about adult ASD include books like Tony Attwood's "The Complete Guide to Asperger's Syndrome" and blogs and vlogs by autistic adults.

Assessing ASD traits in yourself: based on your reading and research, make a list of traits you see in yourself. Talk with one or more trusted persons in your life about your self-assessment. Share a list of ASD traits (female ASD traits) with them. Do they see the same traits that you perceive? Do they see traits you haven't considered?

Looking back at childhood: if you have access to childhood records (baby book, report cards, etc.) or home movies, it can be helpful to look for typical early signs of ASD. If possible, you can also ask your parents or caregivers about specific behaviours. Often, an adult diagnosis will involve answering questions about your childhood, so any information you can gather before an assessment will be helpful.

By the time you've completed your research, you should have a good idea of whether ASD is a good fit for you. Many adults are content with this and choose to self-identify as Aspie or autistic based on their self-discovery process. Others feel the need—or have a specific reason—to seek out a professional diagnosis.

Seeking an adult ASD assessment

If you decide to pursue a professional diagnosis, it's important to find a psychologist, psychiatrist or neuropsychologist experienced in diagnosing adults with ASD. If your child has received a diagnosis, his or her clinician may be able to refer you to someone who does adult assessments. Other options for finding providers who do adult evaluations include: online resources like the Pathfinders for Autism website; recommendations from other autistic adults; parents of autistic children; teaching/research university hospitals; and local non-profit autism service organizations.

Whatever path you take to find someone who can evaluate you, know that it won't likely be a direct route. It's okay to feel like the biggest first step you can manage right now is to make a list of providers to contact. It may take weeks or months to start making those calls and yet more months to commit to meeting with a professional or scheduling an evaluation, especially if you are simultaneously dealing with the demands of being your autistic child's advocate.

Ultimately, most adults find that an autism diagnosis is a positive thing. It provides an explanation for why we've always felt different and is the first step in assembling a toolbox filled with new coping skills and adaptations.

Why Asperger's Hasn't Existed since May 2013

Yes the title sounds odd. Having talked previously about getting an official diagnosis, we are now saying it has gone away. However things are not quite that simple. It simply got reclassified into something else (at least for official purposes).

Let me explain: DSM version 5 (DSM-V) was modified to remove the diagnosis of Asperger's and reclassify those showing those symptoms under the general Autism Spectrum umbrella. The DSM is the d facto tool most doctors use to diagnose individuals, based on their characteristics. The decision to move Asperger's was based on their belief that it would better serve people on the Autism Spectrum.

The problem with this move is that there are people who had been previously diagnosed with Asperger's under DSM-IV but could no longer qualify for a diagnosis under the Autism Spectrum umbrella. This caused a lot of anger for many people in the Asperger's community. They felt the move would make them unrepresented and that they'd simply be absorbed wholesale into the new classification.

There is growing evidence that Asperger's is different to Autism in terms of brain connectivity. In response to the DSM reclassification, there was a research study carried out by Frank Duffy, M.D. He used electroencephalography (EEG) recordings to measure the amount of signalling occurring between brain areas. His findings were that "The ASP population appears to constitute a neurophysiologically identifiable, normally distributed entity within the higher functioning tail of the ASD population distribution." You can read more details about the study at:

http://www.biomedcentral.com/1741-7015/11/175.

Alongside these differences, there are also other differences, such as developmental delays that only become apparent in children with Asperger's as they get older. They typically do not experience the same language delays as children with other elements of Autism Spectrum Disorders.

Some estimates suggest that one third of people who would have previously qualified for a diagnosis of either Autism or Asperger's will no longer fit into either diagnosis category as a result of reclassification. This then has implications for the level of support and insurance-based services that would have previously been available to that individual.

Personally, I find the reclassification trend disturbing. However, the good news is that the European diagnostic classification (the ICD framework) does continue to recognise Asperger's as a separate subgroup.

My hope is that as awareness of the issue is raised, the reclassification will be reversed in the next version of the DSM.

PDD-NOS

In this book, we thought we should include PDD-NOS as this is a slightly alternative diagnosis given to Asperger's in the DSM-IV.

PDD-NOS, or Pervasive Developmental Disorder Not Otherwise Specified, is a type of diagnosis given to individuals on the Autism Spectrum. As a diagnosis, it fits somewhere between Asperger's Syndrome and classic Autism.

Often it is used as a kind of catch all for those that do not fully fit into either category. It can be used as a diagnosis when there is little or no data to support a typical Autism diagnosis with regard to the early part of one's life. Usually classic Autism features developmental issues and social retardation from an early age. With PDD-NOS this information is not always necessary for medical professionals to make an attempt at diagnosis.

The symptoms of PDD-NOS

While PDD-NOS has many of the same characteristics, the major symptoms used to diagnose are:

social impairments

communication impairments

repetitive behaviours.

While these are not the only symptoms, there are other behaviours associated with other conditions that are common with PDD. These include: Autistic Disorder, Asperger's Syndrome, Rett Syndrome and Childhood Disintegrative Disorder.

DSM Criteria

DSM, commonly known as the Diagnostic and Statistical Manual of Mental Disorders, is widely recognised around the world by various psychiatric associations as the standard for clinical diagnosis.

We have included the DSM-IV criteria rather than the later DSM-V one as it (DSM-V) subsequently grouped Asperger's Syndrome together with the more general Autism Spectrum Disorder category and I feel that PDD-NOS still deserves a mention in the old category.

The DSM-IV definition of the category for Pervasive Developmental Disorders Not Otherwise Specified is:

"This category should be used when there is a severe and pervasive impairment in the development of reciprocal social interaction or verbal and nonverbal communication skills, or when stereotyped behavior, interests, and activities are present, but the criteria are not met for a specific pervasive developmental disorder, schizophrenia, schizotypal personality disorder, or avoidant personality disorder. For example, this category includes "atypical autism" – presentations that do not meet the criteria for autistic disorder because of late age of onset, atypical symptomatology, or subthreshold symptomatology, or all of these."

The methodology behind PDD-NOS diagnosis is now becoming a very contentious issue. Many argue that the definition is too weak and that even medical professionals disagree about the correct diagnosis. This could well be a classic example of being placed in a box.

Testing for PDD-NOS

Unlike with Asperger's, there unfortunately does not exist a wide range of testing materials for self-diagnosis. The condition, by its very nature, is difficult to diagnose, as it is, in essence, an umbrella for many conditions within the Autism Spectrum. If you are looking for clues as to the likelihood of having Pervasive Developmental Disorder, we can recommend either using the generic autism quotient test or this experimental assessment on the childbrain website.

If you are concerned whether you may have the condition, we strongly recommend that you visit a medical professional to get more professional advice.

Where is PDD-NOS in DSM-V?

With the advent of DSM-V things became a lot less diverse in all areas of the Autism Spectrum. Classic autism, Asperger's and

PDD-NOS have been rolled into a single Autism Spectrum category.

This is a cause of controversy for many members of the autistic community, who feel that the change in diagnostic criteria is unwelcome. Generic diagnosis such as this never truly represents the true condition of the individual. Some boxes may be ticked but not others, but for the medical professional it does seem easier to give someone a more generic label than to take the time and really understand what is going on.

PDD-NOS resources

There is a neat checklist that can be used for spotting diagnosis on the National Autism Resources website.

Also check out Barbara Quinns book on Pervasive Developmental Disorder, which we highly recommend as a resource guide on the subject.

You can also find a list of recommended books and other resources on our website.

Comorbid Conditions

Comorbid conditions are a set of additional conditions that can occur alongside the primary condition.

In layman's terms this means that people with AS often have other conditions. These may include:

- anxiety disorders
- ADHD
- bipolar Disorder
- bowel disease
- dyspraxia
- dyslexia
- OCD
- Tourette's Syndrome
- sleep disorders.

For anyone reading the list above, don't necessarily be disturbed. Just because you may qualify for an Asperger's diagnosis, it does not mean you have all of these conditions. It's just possible that you have some of them.

Dealing with the diagnosis

Everybody is different when it comes to responding to the diagnosis that they have Asperger's or Autism.

For some, it is a relief because it helps you understand why you are the way you are. You have a reference point and you can understand that there are many people around the world with the same condition. But for many people, accepting the diagnosis is not easy; it can bring memories from the past about occasions when the symptoms were most present. Perhaps from social events, childhood or school.

It's easy to think of ourselves as different and inferior. We don't feel good enough and we often suffer from low self-esteem.

One of the most important things to remember during the period following diagnosis is that Asperger's can be a gift as well as a curse. Yes it's true, sometimes we struggle with life and social skills that are easy for many neurotypical (NT) individuals. However, people with Asperger's Syndrome have many different abilities and qualities. The ability to see and understand the world in different ways with a different perception can add so many gifts to the world.

If you haven't seen the movie about Temple Grandin's struggle with Autism and her subsequent achievements in life, we recommend you do. Not only did Temple find a way to overcome the emotional distress, but she also gained a Ph.D. in animal science and became an internationally recognised speaker in the autistic community. Temple is truly an example to us all.

Without the qualities of Asperger's Syndrome, we wouldn't have the pioneering theory of relativity that was developed by Albert Einstein, or the widespread adoption of the Windows operating system when Bill Gates created Microsoft. It's important to find your contribution to the world, however big or small.

Chapter 3: Aspergers Syndrome

Behavioral Aspect

It is unknown as to what causes Asperger's syndrome. The behavioral aspect of this disorder can render children with Aspergers to behave quite strangely and at times they can even unintentionally make remarks that can be quite rude and painful towards others while being so unaware of their effect from the remarks. This is usually a result of the social disconnect found within children showing signs of Aspergers as well as their lack of imagination that can make it quite easy not to show empathy towards their peers.

Many children with Aspergers grow up to become teens not interested in the latest fads, social norms or conventional ways of thinking. Normally children with Aspergers Syndrome deem themselves to being creative and original thinkers in pursuit of their own goals and interests. Sometimes Aspergers teens can excel in class due to their strong preferences for rules and structure.

Teens with Aspergers can excel in certain fields due to their narrow focus of interest. For example, a teen with Asperger's syndrome may excel greatly in math due to their narrow interest in the subject but struggle in English or History class due to their high disinterest in the field brought on by the sole preoccupation to only be interested in Math.

Parents should be encouraging towards children and teens with Aspergers. Teachers should learn how to respond to students with Asperger's syndrome, but patience is a virtue when dealing with the signs of Asperger's syndrome in children, teens or adults. Every child is different and it is important to establish a safe and trusting environment that can enable the child to reach out if help is sought. Good communication skills can only be learned if the child with Asperger's syndrome feels that they are in a safe and welcoming environment.

MANAGING ASPERGERS SYNDROME BEHAVIOR

For many, the proper diagnosis of Aspergers Syndrome may give rise to the larger problem of how to manage Asperger's syndrome behavior. There are guidelines which can be of assistance in establishing practices designed to help those with Aspergers syndrome develop skills which can lessen the impact of the disorder. These include the following:

Teaching basic skills and concepts should be undertaken with sufferers of Aspergers syndrome in an explicit and deliberate manner with an explanation as to how the parts fit into a larger whole.

Social awareness may need to be instructively promoted rather than intuitively learned, with the focus being given to specific examples of appropriate behavior in discreet situations. A clear emphasis on the difference between the perceptions of a person with Aspergers syndrome as distinct from others should be explained.

Regular visitation of problem-solving techniques, with a focus on providing step-by-step strategies to effectively recognize and deal with common everyday difficulties.

The practice of simultaneously interpreting visual and auditory stimuli should be cultivated with a view to assisting an Aspergers syndrome sufferer in classifying non-verbal behavior, and understanding how that behavior correlates with verbal communication. The implications of eye-contact, non-verbal communication such as hand gestures, facial expression, and obvious body language should be explored. Changes in tone, inflection, and figurative language should be instructed broadly, with increasing specificity over time.

Self-sufficiency may be enhanced by increasing the adaptive skills of those with Aspergers syndrome. Rote learning of specific activities, such as travel or meeting strangers, should be verbally instructed and rehearsed in order that sequential repetition can give rise to learned behavior.

Subsequent reinforcement of those routines should be undertaken by coordination and communication with those responsible for the individual's ongoing care, welfare, and development. Consistency in routine will be a significant factor in its assimilation by the individual into behavior patterns.

Self-awareness and evaluation may need to be independently encouraged to both enable individuals with Aspergers syndrome to perceive appropriate behavior in different social circumstances and to assist with self-esteem when such situations are successfully managed. Again, pre-learned strategies applied in practice to specific examples will compliment the cognitive abilities of those with Aspergers.

The establishment of a 'safety-net' for circumstances where an Aspergers syndrome individual encounters a novel situation should be implemented, with a pre-planned course of action to be undertaken.

The link between certain anxiety provoking experiences and resulting feelings of frustration and depression should be explicitly taught in a 'cause and effect' manner in order to engender within the Aspergers syndrome individual some insight into their own emotions. This can also assist in gaining empathetic response by enabling the individual to have some awareness of the feelings of others. The individual with Aspergers syndrome should be encouraged to monitor their own speech patterns, and be instructed as to the interpretation which others may place upon it.

To assist with age-appropriate communication with their peer group, Aspergers syndrome individuals may be assisted by instructions on how to manage topics of discussion, the importance of topic expansion, closing discussions, and gaining comfort in mutual engagement.

Ultimately, a combination of learned behavior may be explored to establish guidelines to prevent disruptive behavior, assist in more intuitive decision making, and participate in open forms of communication.

The integration of these types of behavior management strategies can be assisted by their coordination both in the home and in the case of children, at school. With proper management and professional assistance, a pro-active and integrated approach to managing Aspergers syndrome behavior can be of both short term and long term benefits to those afflicted by it.

HOW TO COPE ASPERGERS SYNDROME SYMPTOMS?

As many children with autism and other developmental delay disorders, Aspergers syndrome symptoms include having difficulties with social interactions. Children with Aspergers syndrome symptoms usually have the most problems when it comes to the interpretation of nonverbal cues given by other people such as body language and facial expressions.

Forming friendships with other peers can be a difficult task because Aspergers symptoms make it difficult for normal social interactions to take place.

Many people with Aspergers syndrome symptoms have a low desire to share their experiences or interests with other people, for example, if a child with Aspergers syndrome builds a toy, they are more likely to keep the discovery to themselves than to share and brag about it to others such as most children do.

Children with Aspergers have an impressive vocabulary with the exception of course of social skills lacking. Being obsessively interested in a single particular object or subject is yet another defining characteristic of Aspergers syndrome symptoms.

A child with Aspergers syndrome symptoms may choose to become fixated on one single particular subject and be neglectful in taking interest in much else. They can obsessively seek to find advanced information about clocks, maps, and other single topics, but may become quite inflexible even rigid in their habits, routines and rituals.

Odd mannerisms can also arise from children with Aspergers. Hand flapping, as well as other postures, may contribute to making a child with Aspergers to appear clumsy. While growing up, children exhibiting Aspergers symptoms may grow up being seen as "odd", even "eccentric" later on as adults.

Anxiety can at times arise in the case of social interactions, especially in fairly new social situations. Children with Aspergers symptoms can at times have debilitating compulsions due to the introduction of new social situations. There is medical treatment available for anxiety, however, parents, as well as educational facilities, are encouraged to remain patient and to continue the needed social skills training.

ASPERGERS SYMPTOMS ARE TREATABLE

Aspergers is a disorder that is very hard to diagnose because it has variable symptoms and no two people with this disorder act the same. To realize if your child has Aspergers is not an easy thing.

However, there are some symptoms you can try to observe. Asperger's treatment is only possible by managing the symptoms and because the symptoms are varied, every child with Aspergers must be treated according to their own symptoms.

Children with Aspergers have normal cognitive and language development. The problems start when they interact with other children. People with Aspergers Syndrome have difficulties understanding the facial expressions of the others, they don't like eye contact and they don't understand metaphoric statements. They show no physical signs like children with Down syndrome.

Also, no genetic reason or chemical imbalance is found for Aspergers Syndrome. This disorder is considered to be in autism spectrum. This means that it is a kind of autism, differentiating only by its severity or rather its lack of severity. Aspergers is on the high functioning end of autism spectrum. It has very similar characteristics like eye contact problem or repetitive behavior but these symptoms are less severe in children with Asperger's disorder.

There are extensive tests to be able to diagnose Aspergers Syndrome. Once these tests are conducted and a diagnosis is reached, it is very essential to let the child know about the disorder. Children with this disorder see the world from a different window. They are very capable to understand the behaviors of their peers.

Because of their disorder, they are generally isolated and they don't like to be around people. However, this does not mean that they don't like people or they don't want to have friends.

They like people and they would like to have friends but they can't show their feelings and their facial expression usually make people think otherwise. They are extremely intelligent and have a tendency to learn excessive information about a single subject.

When children with this disorder grow up, they usually become very successful people in the areas they choose. The hardest time they live in their childhood and adolescence. To give them the highest possible quality of life their parents must undertake the hard job of protecting them.

Aspergers is a difficult disorder to deal with. However if we compare it to other disorders like Dawn or autistic disorder, the people with Aspergers are luckier. They can have a full, productive life. They can get married, have children and work in a normal environment.

When it is diagnosed early, Asperger's treatment shows more promise. Some symptoms can be alleviated more easily when they don't turn into bad habits. Once the person with Aspergers understands the differences with other people and problems he can face everything becomes easier.

ASPERGER SYNDROME IN ADULTS

Asperger syndrome in adults may be hard for the sufferers and can be a challenge for the people around them as well. Although there is no total cure for this disorder, you can help them cope up with this developmental disorder and live at least a normal life.

Although different persons can exhibit different symptoms, there are signs that are common among sufferers. The most common are difficulty in social interaction and communication and the difficulty to understand body language.

Other signs and symptoms of Asperger syndrome in adults may include their difficulty in abstract thinking, difficulty in empathizing with others, difficulty in understanding other nonverbal communication such as facial expressions, eye contact, and body language. Sufferers of Asperger's syndrome can often be misinterpreted as rude, disrespectful or selfish as they may not be capable of understanding the feelings of the people around them. They may also find it difficult to see a situation in another person's point of view and may not be able to understand appropriate social behavior.

Understand also that people with Asperger syndrome may find it hard to control their emotions and feelings such as anger, anxiety, and depression. Thus, if you are dealing with adults having this disorder, or you may be in a relationship with a person having this disorder, it is best to have tons of patience and understanding and teach them to cope up with such symptoms.

Indeed, Asperger syndrome in adults does not mean they cannot live a normal life, nor they can build good relationships. Adults with this disorder can still lead a good life, get a career, live independently and can get married. However, the challenge in dealing with their behavior may remain. With proper cognitive therapy, support and good education, they will eventually learn to cope up with the symptoms.

In fact, most sufferers of this disorder have average to above average intelligence and they may develop an intense interest on a particular thing or passion like music and math and may excel on it.

If you have a partner with Asperger syndrome, you may also need to have practical and emotional support especially when you already have kids. You have to understand that they find it difficult to understand your feelings and may not be able to support you in what you need so you have to plan everything out and how you can deal with it especially when it comes to parenting.

Finding careers for adults with Asperger syndrome may also require careful selection. Usually, they can get a career which requires visual thinking like careers in design or drafting. They may also get a successful career in music or those that may require good mathematics such as accounting.

To help you deal with Asperger syndrome in adults, it is also helpful to find social training sessions to help the sufferer cope up with his difficulty in social interaction. As a partner, you may also need counseling and guidance in order to deal with this disorder and help you understand your partner well.

LIVING WITH YOUR ADULT CHILD

There are many issues involved in dealing with Asperger's syndrome in adults that you would not necessarily have with other adult children. The issue of readiness to live alone at 18 or 21 is one of them.

Many young adults without neurological disabilities are also living with their parents after graduating from college or high school as well. The press has even given them the name "boomerang kids." Still, living with your adult Asperger's child does have its special challenges. So how do you make sure it works for both of you?

1. Set clear boundaries

To start with, you need to set clear boundaries and rules as to the living situation, and what will be expected of all people in the household. This is a good idea no matter which you are living with. But if you are dealing with an adult child with Asperger's syndrome this has extra importance. Why? Because these adults crave clarity and direction. They completely flounder without it. They do not have the ability to read between the lines and understand what is expected of them. You have to spell it out.

2. Make rules clear

You can save yourself a lot of resentment in the future by making these rules clear ahead of time. Do you want your adult child to help with the chores around the house? Pay rent? Come home by a certain time of night? Limit the number of people they have over? Then tell them in very explicit terms.

Never assume "Oh, a reasonable person would know to put the dishes away without being told" or "Anyone would know it's impolite to have friends over after 11 pm" or whatever it may be -- and then get mad at your child when they break these invisible rules! Common sense is not the strength of a person with Asperger's syndrome. Mostly, they march according to their logic, which makes perfect sense to them. But if you explain to them why you want something a done a certain way or why a certain thing is important to you, then they are perfectly capable of, and usually even eager to, follow the rules.

3. Pay attention to emotional maturity, anxiety, and level of detail

It can be a hard transition for anyone who is leaving the relatively sheltered world of education to whatever comes next. When dealing with Asperger's syndrome in adults, though, going from a structured existence where there were clear goals and ways to accomplish them to an aimless existence in which none of this exists can be very hard. You also have to remember that emotional maturity levels of this age group will be behind typical kids, due to the nature of developmental disabilities.

THE EXPERIENCE OF A YOUNG WOMAN

One young woman reveals the following about her experiences living with her parents after college.

When I lived at my parents' house after college, I was an extremely frustrated person. I had absolutely nothing to do with my time, and no way to get out of the house except for perhaps once a week. I didn't drive, and we lived far from town. I had no control over my life whatsoever.

I would go to my parents for sympathy but they'd just get mad at me. They would go out for dinner, and I'd spend the whole evening resenting that they were able to leave the house and I wasn't. When they'd come home late at night, they'd ask me why I hadn't done the dishes or some other chore, and I'd explode at them about how lucky they were and get mad at them for asking me to help.

It is clear that I had very little emotional maturity at that time. I was drowning in self-pity and didn't even realize it, and it made me a pretty selfish person at that time in my life. I had no way to feel like I had any control over my life, so had no way to get out of it.

I should have been grateful for a place to stay and helped out around the house in return, but no one had made it clear to me that this was what I was expected to do. And I was so deep in my own feelings of remorse for the life I wanted to have that I couldn't see it.

WHAT WOULD HELP THIS SITUATION?

In retrospect, there are a few things that would have made this situation better. When she came home from college, there should have been an in-depth, very detailed explanation of "We're glad to help you out for a little bit and let you stay here, but we expect some things in return. We know the (circumstances of your life that brought you to this place) are very hard, but we still need you to help out." Then list the specific chores she would be responsible for, or at least the specific things she should make a point to look for to see if they needed to be done. Make a chart. Make it visual, make it stick, and most of all, do it at a time when no one is defensive and it's being done out of love rather than resentment.

The method of communication matters for adults with Asperger's Syndrome

Telling someone to do something in a tone of voice that implies you are angry at them will not have the effect you want when dealing with Asperger's syndrome in adults. Adults with Asperger's syndrome are very sensitive to emotion, despite not always being able to display it.

They will pick up on the anger in your tone and be so overwhelmed by it that they will not be able to process what you are saying. The anger is scary to them and makes them go into "survival mode" or at least get very defensive. This takes all their mental energy, and they will totally not remember what you are saying.

Therefore, the mistake will be repeated again and again and again until tensions escalate to unbearable levels. Each party is just trying to do what seems right to them, but both parties fail to see that a lack of proper communication is causing all this resentment. It matters how you communicate.

Be aware of each other's emotions, and pay attention to detail

The level of detail also matters. Telling your adult child to "help around the house more" is a very ambiguous statement. Adults with Asperger's syndrome do not do well with ambiguous statements. Telling them "You should know to do this without us asking" is not helpful either. The feelings of guilt and inadequacy that it creates gets in the way of any helpful message getting across. If they knew to do it, they would be doing it. Most adults with Asperger's syndrome are eager to please.

Be specific on what chores you want to be done when, how many friends is a "few," what time "by night" means, or any other ambiguous statement. You may think "They're so smart, they should know this stuff," but remember, adults with Asperger's syndrome have uneven abilities. They seem very smart in some areas, but can be quite clueless in others.

In most cases, it is not a case of laziness. It's a case of having no idea what one is supposed to do or having too much emotional baggage or anxiety to pay attention to anything but the thoughts in their head. In either case, specific direction can work wonders.

A PARENT'S GUIDE TO ASPERGERS SYNDROME

Kids with Aspergers don't usually share the withdrawn isolation of children with autism and will openly, but often very awkwardly, approach and engage others in social situation. However, their inability to see things through others eyes, and the tendency to go overboard going on and on about their latest obsession, makes them appear selfish, uncaring and insensitive toward other people. This is not necessarily true, they just don't realize how they are perceived or that other people have different interests and feelings than they do.

Many of the children with Aspergers will actually memorize reactions in specific social situations, and recite definitions or examples of emotion, but have a very hard time acting on any of that knowledge in a real situation. Or they will use a rigid application of the specific social rules they have memorized. This can come across as forced eye contact, or the plastered on smile, or laughing at the wrong time. They want friends and do seek out social contact, but over the years their failures in these situations can be devastating.

Kids with Aspergers will sometimes develop very focused and intense interest in something or some activity, that will completely dominate their time and their life, almost to the exclusion of everything else, and they will try to draw whoever they can into the same interest. This is usually seen as normal childhood interest and behavior at first until the obsessive qualities become apparent and problems relating to anything or anyone else starts happening.

Diagnosis

The diagnosis uses the identification of the stereotypical and repetitive behaviors as a central part of how it is diagnosed, but confirmation is done by ruling out anything else that can cause the same symptoms. The motor behaviors that are observed are things like the hand flapping or twisting, complex whole-body movements and walking on tiptoes, repeating the same word or sound over and over again are all typical repetitive behaviors of AS.

Other Issues

Your child may display symptoms that aren't a part of an Aspergers Syndrome diagnosis, but still, affect the child and your whole family. They may have perception difficulties, and problems with fine or gross motor skills, handling emotions, and difficulty sleeping. Many kids on the spectrum (Autism Spectrum) have trouble with SI, or Sensory Integration, and can be overly sensitive or under sensitive to sound light, touch, texture, taste, smell, pain, temperature and other things that stimulate the senses. It may feel soft and nice to you, but to them, it can be actually painful.

Children with Aspergers are more likely to have sleep problems, including difficulty in falling asleep, waking up often at night, and early morning awakenings. Aspergers is also associated with alexithymia, which means having problems identifying and describing one's emotions. My daughter certainly has emotions and feelings, but she has no idea how to describe them or even what they are, or why they are there. Very frustrating.

Special education

Children with AS may require special education services because of their social and behavioral difficulties, although many attend regular education classes. Teens and tween with Aspergers may have difficulty with self-care, organization, and disturbances in a social and romantic relationship. They are usually very smart, but the inability to properly express and the awkwardness of social contact keep many from leaving home as adults, although some gain independence in work and domicile, even marrying and raising a family. Teen and preteen years are hard enough on kids without social difficulties but can be very traumatic for a kid dealing with Aspergers.

Coexisting conditions

Anxiety with AS is very common and is usually centered on change or transition. That is why a consistent schedule is so important. Anxiety and stress during social situations is inevitable because of the constantly changing nature of humans and relationships and situations, there isn't a single right thing to do in every situation. Stress and anxiety will show up usually as a behavior, such as withdrawal, an obsession, hyperactivity, or even aggressive or oppositional behavior.

Depression, and other mood disorders can be the end result of the constant stress and frustration of failing to properly socialize and make friends. Medication and behavior therapy can be used to deal with co-existing problems such as anxiety, depression, inattention, obsessive compulsion, and aggression.

Getting the family involved by helping them to understand what is going on with their child or brother or sister, will have a big impact on the child's future. It will also help with being able to deal with everything that is involved in dealing with a child with Aspergers Syndrome and bring some semblance of normalcy back to the family. Getting help early and involving the whole family as a built-in support system has the best effect on long term outcomes for a child with Aspergers Syndrome.

Chapter 4: Causes Asperger's Syndrome

Research and great studies have not unraveled the root cause of this debilitating disease know s Asperger's syndrome. But since it has been known to affect and enfeeble certain families, then it can categorize as an inherited disease that is carried from one member of family to another. In this case, Asperger's Syndrome is passé from parents to their children.

Is Asperger's Syndrome a Common Disease?

It is through research and much study that Asperger's syndrome has come to be accepted as a unique and lethal disorder. It is because of this that the actual number of children suffering from this condition is yet to be known. But when compared to it autism, its cousin, results show that it is more widespread than autism world over. Study has showed that Asperger's has the capacity to occur up to the tune of four times in male children than in female ones. The diagnosis of Asperger's Syndrome is done in children when they are in the age group of two to six years.

The Diagnosis of Asperger's Syndrome Exams and Tests

Like said earlier Asperger's syndrome is a condition that affects development and the social interaction of an individual. A full diagnosis cannot be fully realized until maximum and conclusive inputs have been put by several parties which include parents, teachers, doctors and caregivers who know the child or the adult very well after a time of observation. When these criteria are met, then one can full declare that the child or person is a victim of Asperger's Syndrome. In summary, the criteria include unusual behavior, interests, social interaction and activities. The diagnosis will also include delay in language development, delay in self-help skills and curiosity in the child about the environment they live in.

When a parent discovers that her child could be suffering from Asperger's Syndrome, he will take the child to hospital. After the doctor has confirmed the presence of the symptoms, he begins by carrying out an evaluation which includes knowing the full medical history of the child. The doctor asks about the child's medical history and its development. Information includes motor development of the child, the child's areas of special interest, its language, and the social interactions. The doctor will go further and inquire about the conditions of the mother's during pregnancy and more so the child's family medical history and its motor skills. The child's test and assessment on his personality may also be done.

These tests are vital since they assist the doctor in finding out whether the child's situation is Asperger's Syndrome related. It is out of these results that the care provider may advice the parent to take their child to a specialist for further testing. These tests include intellectual function, and the evaluation of learning styles. The child may be subjected to an IQ test or Intelligence Quotient. Formal language and speech are further evaluated while the child may be tested to find how well he understands the language and its use in communication of the aforesaid ideas. The doctor may also test the child on whether he understands the different forms of communication which includes non-literal language skills and nonverbal types of communication. The child may be tested on whether has understands metaphors and humor in his communication. The doctor will thus listen keenly to the child's pitch, volume, stress levels of the child. In psychiatrically tests, the doctor will examine the child's family and his peer interactions and his reactions to new state of affairs. He will also be tested on his ability to comprehend the feelings of different people. And the different forms of indirect communication which includes teasing and also sarcasm. The doctor may go further and observe the child's behavior at school and at home. But the doctor will go further and test for conditions that cause depression and even anxiety in the child which go hand in hand with people who suffer from Asperger's syndrome. The doctor will not conclude his tests until sees that the child's conditions meet the criteria that have been published by the American Psychiatric Association's in the Diagnostic and Statistical Manual of Mental Disorders (DSM-5).

He will then continue to carry out a neurological and physical test. Majority of people and children with Asperger's will show evidence of dyspraxia and muscle tone or he could be having the two coordination issues. Tests to verify that a child or a person has this condition may not have real tests like for a person suffering from Diabetes. But even then, the doctor may make do with various tests which include X-rays and even blood tests. The doctor can tell and deduce whether a physical disorder could be the major of this condition in the person or child.

But incase the doctor does not find any of these disorders; he may recommend that the child be taken to a specialist who is well versed in childhood development challenges. But not every medic can handle this condition and so again he may be referred to a child or adult psychiatrist doctor may also deem it fit to refer the child to a psychologist. He may also refer the child to a pediatric neurologist or a developmental-behavioral pediatrician. Depending on the condition, he may refer the child to any other health professional who well versed in the diagnosis and treatment of Asperger's syndrome. Other factors may come into play when this diagnosis is taking place. The level of the child's development plus the doctor's observance of the child's behavior and speech are considered. The doctor may go further in his tests which may include her ability to socialize and play with the rest of his friends. But this diagnosis cannot end without the parents, close friends and teachers who know the child well's input on the child's symptoms.

Is Asperger's Syndrome Treatable?

Treatment designed to meet individual needs and available family resources. Specific treatments are based on symptoms. For Asperger's syndrome, a parent should by all means help his child to, interact with the rest of the people and be able to fit in society. It is a major preparation in helping the child grows in life.

Like said earlier, the causes of this disease are yet to be established and therefore its cure is yet to be known. But that notwithstanding, its treatment has been known to improve the functioning and reduce some unwanted behaviors while at the same time improve the functioning of the body. The above statement may provoke the question on how this treatment is carried out. And so the following combination of treatment has been known to improve the wellbeing of the patient. Special education is a system that is formulated to address the child suffering from Asperger's Syndrome unique and diverse educational needs.

Behavioral modification is a system and strategy that is tailored to support positive behavior in a child suffering from Asperger's Syndrome and help reduce their behavioral problems.

Speech, occupational or physical therapy is systems made to help increase a child who has Asperger's Syndrome's functional capabilities. But social skills therapies are programs that are run by psychologists, speech pathologist, counselors and social workers. They are in valuable therapies tailored to build the social skills and abilities of these children with Asperger's Syndrome to read both non-verbal and verbal cues that are often in children and adults suffering from Asperger's.

And finally there is the place of medication in the treatment of people with Asperger's Syndrome. Since this condition still under research, medication to inhibit it is yet to be found. But even then, medications are available that help treat Asperger's syndrome. But these drugs are only used in the treatment of particular symptoms which include depression hyperactivity, anxiety and neurotic behavior.

Chapter 5: Treatment Options And Interventions

Early diagnosis and intervention for developmental disorders such as Autism or Asperger's syndrome is crucial. This is because individuals who experience a developmental delay because of their condition significantly harm the quality of their life. The main advantage of an early diagnosis and intervention is that it minimizes the delays in development allowing the person to properly cope and reach normal milestones in the particular stages of his or her life.

For instance, a person who receives the proper treatment during the early stages of the development of the disorder allows him to have better communication and social skills. Repetitive and unwanted behaviors are also addressed and managed properly. This allows him to readily control and cope with his challenging behaviors. He is also given the opportunity to learn and develop basic activities needed for daily living. When he is supported and treated sooner, he is more likely to learn and practice independent living. His fine motor skills and physical coordination will also be more advanced when he is able to practice them early on.

The treatment options and interventions for Asperger's syndrome range from those that are backed by research and evidence to those that rely on anecdotal evidence. Of course, experts recommend the use of evidence-based treatment instead of the others because of its proven effectiveness when it comes to treating the symptoms of the disorder. However, this does not mean that other approaches that are not backed up by rigorous research should not be considered. Some evidence-based treatments may still not be applicable to everyone. There may be cases wherein individuals with Asperger's find treatments based on word-of-mouth more effective. This is why careful research and proper procedures must still be done to determine the interventions that will work for the patient.

Traditional Treatment Options

Asperger's Syndrome is an irreversible condition. But it can be managed with therapies and strategies, which can further improve functions, thinking abilities, perception and behaviors. The typical interventions for Asperger's include social skills training, cognitive behavioral therapy, occupational therapy, speech therapy as well as training and support for parents and caregivers.

a. Behavioral Interventions

Applied Behavior Analysis

Applied Behavioral Analysis (ABA) is a technique used to analyze and modify behavior. It is found to be an effective way of treating Autism because of its ability to improve behavior by monitoring the response of an individual to a few environmental modifications. In other words, this treatment method involves the careful observation, measurement and analysis of the relationship between an individual's behavior and environment.

ABC Model is the first step in the Applied Behavior Analysis. Through this model, the therapist or caregiver can analyze the behavior of the person with Asperger's. In this approach, ABC stands for Antecedent, Behavior, and Consequence. The antecedent is considered to be the direct appeal for the patient to act in a certain way. Then, behavior means the response of the individual to the said command (this could either be successful, noncompliance, or no response). Lastly, consequence is the response of the therapist or caregiver to the behavior of the individual.

If you want to help your child or anyone with Asperger's syndrome you can employ some of the most common techniques that are used in ABA. These include:

☐Shaping

Shaping simply means the gradual process of modifying and managing challenging behaviors. Therapists and caregivers use this technique by immediately intervening and correcting unwanted behavior. For instance, if a child with Asperger's keeps on hitting his head, hold his hand when he attempts to hit himself and instead turn it into a stroking motion.

☐ Chaining

Chaining is the technique wherein complicated tasks are broken down into small, more manageable partitions. This is similar to breaking down a long method into a step-by-step procedure.

☐ Reinforcement

Reinforcement is simply the process of responding in a certain way to increase the frequency of a desired behavior. The response of the therapist or caregiver depends on the child's behavior as well as the task's level of difficulty. It is rational to reinforce more complicated tasks heavily and easy tasks less heavily. Some examples of reinforcements include activities that the child finds interesting, special treats, stickers, tokens, or free time.

Early Intensive Behavioral Intervention

The Early Intensive Behavioral Intervention or EIBI is quite similar with the methods used in the Applied Behavior Analysis. It also includes the evaluation of the patient's current abilities, strengths, and weaknesses. Their skills are also developed and improved through the use of positive reinforcement. The full cooperation and participation of the therapist and caregiver must be apparent in order for this approach to work.

b. Biomedical Interventions

The usual approach to biomedical interventions involves the intake of certain medications, supplements, and the adherence to a strict diet.

Medication

Medications are often used to reduce the effects of the symptoms found in certain disorders such as ADHD, OCD, depression, and anxiety. Medication is provided to people with these conditions somehow reduce and manage their manifestation. Experts discourage the use of medication when the patients are still physically and cognitively developing. The most common medications prescribed to relieve symptoms of Asperger's Syndrome are Aripiprazole to reduce irritability; Guanfacine, Olanzapine, and Naltrexone to reduce hyperactivity; Selective Serotonin Reuptake Inhibitors (SSRIs) to reduce repetitive behaviors; and Risperidone to reduce agitation and insomnia.

Diet

Proponents of this approach claim that proper nutrition and some diet restrictions can significantly improve the behavior of people with Autism or Asperger's syndrome. Some parents that have restricted their child's diet by removing foods with casein and gluten report that their child had developed a general positive mood. They have also observed that their child showed more eye contact and less aggression.

Vitamins

The use of vitamin B to treat Autism was based on the theory that was formulated back in the 1960's. This theory claimed that vitamin deficiency is a viable cause for the emergence of certain psychiatric disorders. This is why some parents are open to the use of high doses of vitamin B6 to combat the symptoms of Asperger's.

c. Developmental Interventions

Developmental Social-Pragmatic model

The Developmental Social Pragmatic model seeks to help an individual with Asperger's improve his communicative abilities. It focuses on identifying the current skills of the individual then work from there. It strives to help a person with Asperger's initiate a conversation, form friendships and establish deep relationships with other people. This is done by allowing the child to mingle and initiate an interaction based on his own interests. The strategies used in this approach include the provision of meaningful activities that foster spontaneous social communication. Therapists and caregivers who use this approach encourage their child to initiate contact. They also modify the environment of the child in ways that encourage social interaction.

Relationship Development Intervention

The goal of Relationship Development Intervention (RDI) is to promote the social skills and emotional abilities of people that fall under the Autism Spectrum. It seeks to motivate the individual to engage in social interactions and relationships. Dr. Steven Gustein, the developer of this approach, believes that "individuals on the autism spectrum can participate in authentic emotional relationships if they are exposed to them in a gradual, systematic way". This approach is fairly easy to implement. If you want to start using RDI to build your loved ones social connection, you start talking to them by asking a few questions and waiting for their response. You can also create subtle disruptions to their daily routine to help them develop coping skills. Furthermore, you can engage in fun and productive activities that both of you find interesting. Doing so would allow you to gain shared fun experiences that you can talk about.

d. Sensory Integration Therapy

People with Asperger's syndrome typically experience problems with their sensory perception. This is why it is important for caregivers to provide them the special care and attention that they need. Individuals who suffer from sensory problems such as hypersensitivity and hyposensitivity have certain needs that need to be addressed.

Sensory Integration Therapy

Sensory Integration Therapy basically works by providing the child with just the right stimulation to challenge his senses. This would encourage him to adapt to the situation and actively participate to the fun activities that are presented to him. This would cause them to develop a heightened tolerance to the activities that they normally would have no interest in.

To find out which activities are ideal for your child, you need to determine if he or she has a heightened or lowered sensitivity. You can experiment with the stimulation of your child's senses by being mindful of their preferences when it comes to their sense of touch, sight, and hearing.

Occupational, Auditory, & Visual Therapy

The goal of occupational therapy is to help an individual function in daily life activities independently. Through this approach, individuals with Autism are more able to develop and improve their fine motor, social, play, and coping skills. Other therapies focus on developing an individual's sensory perceptions. There are therapies that are specifically formulated to target, address and manage problems with hearing and vision.

Things to Remember:

☐ There are therapies and strategies that can help them improve their social skills, communication skills, and behavior.

☐ Communication skills training and cognitive behavioral training are being provided.

☐ Pediatricians along with psychiatrists can perform an in depth-assessment for this condition.

☐ Medications may be prescribed, but these medications do not remove the disorder. Such medications merely alleviate the symptoms experienced by the person. These medications are palliative treatments.

☐ Medications include Guanfacine, Olanzapine, Selective Serotonin Reuptake Inhibitors (SSRIs),and Risperidone.

☐ Support groups should be readily available.

☐ Support groups include family, relatives, friends, and co-workers. Even doctors and teachers are considered part of their support network that can help the person cope with the difficulties of having Asperger's Syndrome.

☐ Support groups are there to guide, comfort, and make them feel that they can talk to you and count on you.

☐ Support group can let them feel they are not alone

Chapter 6: Facts And Myths About Asperger's Syndrome

Loved ones that recently find out that their relative, friend, or special someone has Asperger's Syndrome usually try too hard in order for them to know and understand the condition better. It is also typical for any concerned loved one to get overwhelmed with information, case studies, or treatment options while they are researching about how they can support and cope with Asperger's. Although the condition has been discovered and heavily researched ever since it was first described by Hans Asperger, a lot of myths and misunderstandings still exist about it. As someone who knows a person with Asperger's you need to be able to distinguish the facts from fiction to provide the support and guidance they need.

Myth 1: He or she will grow out of it

Myths about the potential causes of this condition have been also discussed. First, some people say that children with Asperger's Syndrome will eventually grow out of it. Just like with Attention Deficit Hyperactivity Disorder, there's a prevalent myth that Asperger's Syndrome is strictly a childhood disorder that disappears after the young adulthood stage. But Asperger's Syndrome is known to be a lifelong condition. The symptoms get better with therapies, strategies and medical management, but technically, it never goes away.

Myth 2: It is rare for a person with Asperger's to get married

Another myth is that some adults with Asperger's Syndrome don't get married. As per Bryna Siegel, the Autism Clinic director at the University of California, San Francisco, it is rare that you would see a parent with Asperger's Syndrome. This myth stems from a belief that people with Asperger's are more familiar with short-lived marriages and may lack the ability to maintain a life-long relationship due to their difficulties with social interaction and in establishing a relationship. Though people with this condition may come off as shy and perceive to lack the skilled required in a long-term romantic relationship, there are definitely treatments out there to improve social skills, so to have this belief about Asperger's is a false representation.

Myth 3: Having Asperger's Syndrome automatically means that he or she has social phobia

In addition, adults with Asperger's Syndrome are believed to have a social phobia. This myth is also probably due to their difficulty in social interactions. However, according to Dr. Valerie Gaus, a licensed clinical psychologist centered in New York, a person with a social phobia knows how to communicate and interact with other people, but they are not using those skills because they are afraid it may lead to a poor outcome. They have fear of rejection. This is one of self-preservation.

Myth 4: People with Asperger's are purposely insensitive

Another myth about adults with Asperger's Syndrome is that they are aloof and uninterested in others. This may be because they are not aware of the social conventions in society. With this in mind, sometimes they may talk in a very loud tone of voice in areas where being quiet is permitted, say in a library. It may seem that they are unaware of how to show empathy and they lack the proper response in a conversation. Some people may think that people exhibiting this aloofness to empathy and proper responses in conversation don't care, but the truth is that they just don't know how and what to say.

Myth 5: Everyone with Asperger's is a genius

Like everybody else, the intelligence of people with Asperger's still varies. They usually fall on the extreme ends of the spectrum; either below normal or above average intelligence.

People assume that everyone with Asperger's is brilliant because of their extensive knowledge about a certain topic.

They fail to take into account the fact that individuals with Asperger's have the capability to fixate on something and be very passionate about their interests.

It would be unhealthy to assume and expect too much from your loved one with Asperger's especially when he or she belongs to the lower end of the spectrum. The bottom line is that you should never stop expecting something good for your loved one, but you should also not pressure them too much when it comes to honing and developing their abilities.

Myth 6: I should be able to give my child or loved one a normal life

Some parents believe that as primary caregivers, they should be able to let their child or loved one live a "normal" life. This is a common misconception because a lot of people are striving to make their loved one with Asperger's or Autism think and act like a "normal person". The goal of primary caregivers should be to guide and support their loved one live more independently instead of trying so hard to make them "normal".

Although having Asperger's can make simple things seem more complicated and challenging, they are still doable with the proper mindset and attitude. In order to help your child or loved one live and experience life more by exposing him to typical activities, proper planning and a whole lot of patience and understanding is needed.

Myth 7: I need to find the root cause of his condition

Since Asperger's is considered a disorder, it is typical for anyone to try and determine the root cause of the problem for its prevention and cure. Unfortunately, Asperger's and other forms of Autism are not caused by a single factor. In fact, it is said that the interplay of biological and environmental factors contribute to the emergence of this condition. Instead of using your time and resources on trying to find out the root cause as to why your loved one developed Asperger's syndrome, you should focus on formulating strategies to help him or her function better and eventually live more independently.

Now that we have addressed some of the most common misconceptions that people have about Asperger's, let us focus on the positive side of the condition that are definitely worth celebrating.

Fact 1: They can focus and pay a lot more attention to details

When compared with other people, individuals diagnosed with Asperger's usually show incredible skills when it comes observing, memorizing or making sense of certain things. This is because their attention is more attuned to certain objects or events especially when it falls under their area of interest.

Fact 2: They hardly ever lie

It is typical for people with Asperger's to be blunt and direct to the point because they often interpret things literally. In general, they also tend to adhere to the rules that are set for them to follow.

Fact 3: They do not give in to peer pressure

Unlike others, people with Asperger's are usually not into keeping up with the latest trends and fads. Their decisions are not easily affected by the expectations of the people around them. They usually determine their choices based on the things that they are truly passionate about. They can always stay true to themselves because they do not worry about fitting in.

Fact 4: People with Asperger's Syndrome are passionate

Although the personalities and characteristics of people with Asperger's still vary, many people with this condition become passionate about certain things. They could show a fervent interest in certain topics such as geology, history or mathematics.

Chapter 7: Affecting The Communication Of A Person With As

Take on the role of a helper and teacher
This is one of the ways in which you can affect the communication of a child. When the child is unable to communicate their needs it is tempting to help them by constantly doing things for them. For example, fetching their shoes and tying their shoelaces. However, by doing this the opportunities for the child to show that they can do such things for themselves are reduced. When the child is at the Own Agenda Stage it is particularly difficult to decipher how much to do for the child. In this instance it is appropriate to ask the child if they need help, wait and then ask a second time before offering the help.

Instead of letting the child do their own thing, encourage them to do things with others

It is tempting to believe that the child is merely showing their independence when they show no interest in interacting with the adult. However, it is important that the child does learn to interact and is not just left to own their devices. In this instance the key is to persevere with joining in with whatever activity the child is engaged in, whether this is playing with a piece of string or taking toys in and out of the toy box. If the child shows anger and aggression when this is tried, still persevere. Anger is a type of interaction and is better than no interaction at all. As this interaction is continued with the child they may begin to realize in time that interaction with another person can be fun.

Slow down the pace and give the child a chance to communicate

Caring for a child with AS can be hard work and time consuming. There is often the temptation to rush the child when they are performing daily tasks such as eating breakfast and getting dressed. A child with AS will benefit from an extra few minutes when engaged in these tasks to help them understand what is happening around them and to think about what they can say during these activities.

When playing with the child take on the role of a partner rather than a leader

As the child becomes more capable at communicating, they need less direction. If they are given too many questions and suggestions it can become difficult for them to initiate their own conversations. It is important to follow the child's lead and respond to what they do.

Present the child with feedback

It is important to reward the child when they attempt to understand and communicate. By doing this you can increase the likelihood that they will try and do it again. By using simple descriptive praise that comment on what the child has achieved, the child can make a connection between their own actions and your specific words.

Giving the child with AS a reason to communicate

If the child with AS has no difficulty getting what they want, they will have no reason to communicate and interact. Therefore, on many occasions the adult will need to engineer a situation in order to create a communicative opportunity for the child and encourage interaction.

Encouraging requests

This can be achieved by placing the child's favorite toy/food/video in a place where the child can see it but is unable to reach it, for example, a high shelf. Alternatively, place the child's favorite object in a container, which the child finds difficult to open such as an old ice-cream tub or an old jam jar. This will encourage the child to ask for help and result in an interaction between adult and child.

Give the child a toy that is difficult to operate

Windup toys and games that need to be squeezed to make them work will be difficult for the child to operate alone but will also interest the child. Once the child has been given the toy/game, allow them some time to establish how to use it.

When the child becomes frustrated at their inability to work the toy/game, the adult can step in and help them. Examples of this type of toy include jack-in-the boxes, spinning tops and music boxes.

Give the child a toy that is high interest

Balloons and bubbles are high interest toys and can be easily adapted to involve two people. Simple games such as blowing up a balloon and then letting it go so that it flies up in the air may appeal to the child. Blowing up the balloon part away and waiting for a response from the child before blowing it up to its full capacity is also a clever way to enhance interaction between adult and child. A similar thing can be achieved with bubbles – blow a few bubbles towards the child, once their attention has been captured, close the container and wait for a response from them before you blow more.

Give things to the child gradually

If the child is given everything that they want they will have no reason to ask the adult for anything else. By staggering how much food/how many toys are given to the child they are provided with opportunities to interact by expressing their wants and needs. For example, if the child wants a biscuit, break it into small pieces, initially give them one piece and then gradually give them more once they have communicated a request for it.

Let the child decide when to end an activity

Once the child is engaged in an activity with the adult, carry on with that activity until the child indicates that they have had enough. Look out for facial grimaces or the child pushing away the activity. This way, the child is forced to communicate that they are ready to finish the activity. If the child does not use language to indicate they have finished, accompany their form of communication with words such as had enough and stop to encourage their language development.

Increasing interaction by following the child's lead

Following the child's lead rather than directing them will enable them to learn to communicate while they do things with another person, hence increasing their interaction. The child that leads is more likely to pay attention to the activity, more likely to focus on the same thing as the adult and will learn how to make choices for themselves.

When following the child's lead it is beneficial to be in position where the adult is face-to-face with the child, this way the adult can easily observe what it is that the child is interested in. It will also help the child to make eye contact, something that can often be difficult for the child with an ASD. Being same level with the child will ensure that they are in a position to see the variety of facial expressions that are used in communication. A child will often fail to pick up on these non-verbal communicative behaviors during conversation; therefore, it is important to draw attention to them where possible. It is hoped that the child will eventually become used to the adult playing with them at their level and begin to anticipate their presence, fetching them if they are not there.

Imitating the child's actions and words will help the child become involved in two-way interactions. If the child bangs the spoon on the table, and the adult does the same, it is likely that the child will pay attention to the adult. This idea can also be used with sounds that the child makes or with the child's sensory behaviors, for example, hand flapping and spinning. Once the child has established that the adult is imitating her actions, they may begin to imitate back. This creates the opportunity for the adult to add something new to the exchange for the child to duplicate.

When the child is disinterested in playing with any of the toys presented, or prefers to line toys up rather than play with them, there are still communication and interaction opportunities available. For example, if the child is lining up their cars in rows, the adult can join in the activity by handling the child the cars one by one. This way, the adult plays a part in the game and the child has to include them in what they are doing. If the child is only interested in throwing the toys on the floor, the adult could use a basket to collect them before giving them back to them, thus establishing a pattern of interaction and communication with the child.

Chapter 8: The Future Is Bright

When you have a loved one who is AS-challenged, he is different from others. Since you know he has developmental incapacities, it is normal for you to worry about what the future may hold for him.

Will he ever get better? Will he ever be capable to live independently? What happens when he's older?

What you can expect

The first thing you must expect: an Aspie will always be an Aspie. There is no cure for AS so there is no point in hoping for AS to go away. The other thing you must expect is that, given the proper support, treatment, and therapy, Aspies tend to get better over time.

Personality-wise, expect an Aspie to remain seemingly emotionally detached. Learn not to feel bad when he seems to be neglecting you or your feelings. Accept that he is not deliberately ignoring you, he just can become overly focused at what he does.

He will always be blatantly honest and seemingly judgmental about your faults and mistakes. Know that he does not mean to put you down. It just so happens that he is wired to want to fix things because he wants everything to be perfect, including you. When you don't appreciate 'getting fixed', tell him—it's the only reason for him to know and to understand.

All the things he does as a child with AS, he will continue to manifest into adulthood. With proper guidance and treatment, however, you can expect to see improvements.

Aspies, in general, tend to live full lives. Although, co-morbid conditions like anxiety and depression, are likely to threaten this possibility.

The future holds promises for an Aspie

Will your loved one with AS ever be independent and capable of living on his own? Will he ever be able to build lasting, meaningful relationships with other people? Will he ever experience a first love and build his own family?

Trust that Aspies have done it before, and more are becoming capable of doing so with little help from families and friends. Successful Aspies include: film actor and writer, Dan Aykroyd; "Britain's Got Talent" sensation, Susan Boyle; and, author and food animal systems handling designer, Temple Grandin, who, in 2010, was also named by Time Magazine as one of the 100 most influential people in the world.

Many Aspies tend to experience major improvements in their condition, with the proper treatment, care, and support. Many eventually become capable of attending regular schools and universities, and eventually become successful doing mainstream jobs. Many eventually move out of their parents' homes and live on their own.

Do Aspies get married? Absolutely! As a matter of fact, AS tends to run in families. Relationships and marriages involving Aspies will continue to become challenging, and it will remain hurtful if the Aspie's loved ones continue to evaluate an Aspie based on societal norms. Unless an Aspie's loved ones become more capable of understanding his world, they will be dissatisfied in their relationships with an Aspie.

Continuing commitment

Loving and accepting an Aspie for everything that he is and everything that he isn't must become a continuing commitment of everyone around him that love him and care for him.

Support is something your Aspie loved one will need from birth until well into adulthood. Although, the kind and intensity of support needed may become different and tend to improve over time, if and when the proper interventions are set early on.

Still, there can be many hardships along the way which may never go away but, the situation may be altered only when you start seeing what your Aspie loved one says and does from a different angle. That is, never expect an Aspie to say or do things in a relationship that can only be expected when both parties are typical, non-AS-challenged individuals.

Be certain about it: you, more often than he ever will, will have to make adjustments to accommodate the emotional limitations of your Aspie loved one. So, expect to give more than you can ever take.

Advances in AS treatment

The AS treatment strategy has remained quite the same throughout the past few decades: it has always been a combination of medication and therapies. However, there is no one menu of treatment that applies for all Aspies.

Each Aspie is unique. Each one has to deal with a different set of strengths and limitations that call for different interventions. Therapies are introduced to improve limitations in speech, motor skills, behavior, and cognition. These are designed to help Aspies cope with their limitations. Common problems with focus are dealt with often by encouraging Aspies to take up an interest and hobby which, more often than not, Aspies tend to excel in.

Medication drugs for Aspies have seen some major advances throughout the years. Today, some of the medications available for Aspies include: psychostimulants to address problems with focusing and hyperactivity; selective serotonin reuptake inhibitors (SSRIs) to address obsessive and compulsive tendencies; mood stabilizers to help manage behavior and emotions; and, SSRIs and antidepressants to help treat anxiety.

Despite the more sophisticated treatment alternatives available for Aspies today, one ingredient has remained essential to an Aspie's betterment: the love, acceptance, and support of families and friends.

You do not need to lead an Aspie. He will know what he needs and is a natural survivor. Rather than focusing on how you can intervene in his condition, pay attention to what he's telling you---he is wired for survival so he will know what he needs, when he needs it most. Let your Aspie lead the way.

Chapter 9: Effects Of The Syndrome On Speech And Language

In some cultures, to indicate that something is extremely obvious, they use the following joke:

"What meows on the roof and is not a dog that also learns foreign languages?"

It is obvious that the answer to this question is "a cat." In the case of Asperger's, unfortunately, the aspie may be the dog that tries to learn foreign languages. As stated in relevant studies, in many cases linguistic communication for people with AS is an attempt at mimicry without any understanding of the underlying nuances.

The concept of language is the vocal expression of meanings and feelings. The correct use of language means that the person who is speaking interprets the meanings and feelings of his own brain and matches them to the appropriate words in an orderly fashion.

Aspies usually do not experience delays in the acquisition of language skills, and their speech patterns are quite normal. But they may **seem** to be atypical, in that they incorporate any or all of the following in their use of language:

Verbosity

Pedantism

Literal interpretation

Lack of nuance comprehension

Abrupt transitions

Use of metaphors that make sense only to the speaker

Formal or idiosyncratic speech

This atypical use of language most often results from problems in the auditory perception of the aspie. While the sounds will reach the brain, due to the abnormalities of the brain functions, the individual will have difficulty in correctly interpreting and understanding the sounds he or she hears, especially those that pertain to speech. These auditory perception deficits may also result in peculiar uses of loudness, pitch, prosody, intonation and rhythms of speech patterns.

For an accurate diagnosis of the syndrome, three aspects are needed: prosody that is poor, circumstantial and tangential speech, and marked verbosity. These are indicated by the following factors:

Limited range of intonation

Unusually fast, jerky and loud speech

Speech that may sound incoherent

Monologues on topics that result in the boredom of the listener

Speech that fails to provide context for comments

Speech that fails to suppress internal thoughts

Failure to understand if the listener is interested in the topic or not

Failure to understand if the listener is engaged in the conversation

Failure to conclude or make a point

Disregard of the listener's attempts to elaborate on the topic

Disregard of the listener's attempts to change the topic

Hans Asperger called the children under his care "little professors." This was due to their literal usage of language. Aspies seem to have difficulty in understanding and using **figurative speech.** Consequently, expressions of humor, irony, sarcasm and teasing seem not only to escape them completely, but also to insult them.

Especially in the case of humor, aspies may understand the cognitive basis but cannot understand the concept of humor being used as a means to share enjoyment with other people. Strangely, while the evidence for the lack of humor appreciation is strong, there have been reports of humor in aspies that challenge some of the theories about the psychological status of the people that exhibit the symptoms of AS.

Sometimes aspies will display **echolalia**. The term is the same as **echologia** or **echophrasia**. This is the automatic or delayed repetition of speech that the aspie hears from another person. The relevant studies conducted in the 1980s, theorized that they do this in an attempt to communicate through imitative behavior.

The practice can be considered an attempt at the superficial processing of linguistic skills or at the deeper level processing of contextual information. It may also be an attempt to learn.

When an aspie repeats a phrase he or she has heard on the TV or radio, a favorite script or a parental instruction, he or she may be attempting to process this information for the purpose of understanding the meanings and thus becoming able to use them later on in discussions.

While this intention may work and the aspie may memorize the phrase, he or she may not understand under which circumstances and context this phrase is to be used, and therefore, use it out of context. This falls under the category of incoherent speech.

Echolalia has resulted in disputes and debates among the scientific community. For scientists like **Uta Frith, Prizant** and others, echolalia is evidence of Gestalt processing. The term **Gestalt** belongs to the Berlin School of Psychology and indicates an attempt to separate, acquire and keep perceptions of meaning out of an apparently chaotic world.

On the other hand, **Tager-Flusberg** and **Calkins** conducted a study in 1990 on the acquisition of grammar by autistic children which showed that echolalia did not actually facilitate or contribute in any way to the grammatical development of people with AS.

Corresponding to echolalia, many aspies use **echopraxia**. Just like echolalia mimics sounds, echopraxia mimics body and hand motions and gestures. Both echolalia and echopraxia are imitated without explicit awareness of what actually is meant and why.

If these imitative behaviors are performed by aspies on their own they may mean nothing. But if they are conducted within the guidelines of behavioral therapies, they may have a very positive result. According to the stipulations of the study of **Ganos et al.** in 2012, both echolalia and echopraxia are useful, normal and necessary components for teaching social skills. As the study puts it:

"The imitating observer acquires new behaviors by reenacting previously shown motor or vocal patterns."

The distinction between actually learning and simply imitating cannot be made until the child reaches the age of three, when he or she starts to develop the ability to self-regulate.

It is rather evident from all the relevant studies that the problems of speech and language are derived from problems in perception. When the normal people use the word "window," they could mean "window of opportunity." The aspie does not comprehend this notion. When he or she uses the word "window," he or she means it literally.

On the other hand, this does not mean that all the people with AS have linguistic problems. On the contrary, it has been well documented that children with AS may have unusually sophisticated vocabularies and that their use of language is advanced for their ages.

This is where behavioral therapies focus. They teach the nuances and other meanings of words so that the aspie may acquire broader knowledge of language and, therefore, become able to better integrate socially.

Effects of the Syndrome on Motor and Sensory Perception

The issue of physical clumsiness has been repeatedly mentioned in the previous chapters. It's time to elaborate on how Asperger's affects the motor and sensory perceptions of an individual.

The first thing to mention at this point is that motor and sensory perception problems may be independent of the diagnosis. They do affect the individual that suffers from the syndrome and their family, but they are not particularly sought out when the diagnosis is being made.

Motor perception is actually an improper term scientifically. The proper term is **perceptual motor development** and is defined as a person's ability to receive, understand and respond to information provided by the five senses of the human body. An aspie may have difficulty or inability in any of the three components of this definition. The clinical evidence so far indicates that the majority of aspies fail to understand what their minds are receiving, resulting in an inability to provide an appropriate response.

Sensory perception is the information received by a stimulus to any of the five senses of the body (touching, smelling, hearing, seeing, tasting) and the transmission of this information through the nervous system to the brain, where it will be processed by the motor perception. Clinical evidence shows that unless there is another medical condition in co-existence (myopia, reduced hearing, deaf-muteness, etc.), there are no significant problems in the way the senses work in people with AS.

Motor and sensory perception defects pertain to motor skills, sleep and emotions. Actually the term **defects** is incorrect, as aspies, in most cases, have such excellent visual and auditory perception that even the slightest of changes in a familiar environment is immediately noticed. Aspies' difficulties lie mostly in tasks that need a combination of visual and spatial perception and/or auditory and visual memory.

The auditory and visual memories especially present a problem. The term **memory** implies that something is stored in the brain to be accessed and used again at a later time. Visual memory of a fire, for example, recalls that if one gets too close to the flame, one will be burned. Auditory memory of an object maintains that if one scratches a specific object with a piece of metal, the resulting sound will be thoroughly unpleasant.

Aspies may be unusually perceptive to sound, light and other stimuli. On the other hand, they might also be totally insensitive to the exact same stimuli. The clinical evidence so far seems to be more in support of the hypothesis of decreased responsiveness to sensory input almost to the point of no reaction at all, even though there have been several recorded cases of exactly the opposite.

But no matter how acute their perception of sound and light may be, it does them no good if they cannot correlate an image or a sound with a situation. And that may be unnecessary if the sensation produced is positive or pleasant. But what happens if the sensation is negative? They are forced to relive the same unpleasant experience again and again unless there is an intervention.

A most worrying issue in the motor and sensory perception, directly linked to the problems of auditory and visual memory, is that there may not be any **flight-or-fight** mechanism. This is the mechanism that makes people respond to danger either by standing and fighting or by fleeing, and is one of the most vital physiological defensive mechanisms in humans.

Aspies may just stand there and do nothing at all when an attack or other harmful event occurs or when a threat to survival is present. This is one of the main reasons that they are subject to manipulation, victimization and bullying and that constant supervision is required.

The flight-or-fight mechanism depends upon discharges of the sympathetic nervous system. Hormones like estrogen and testosterone and neurotransmitters like dopamine and serotonin are released throughout the human body for the purpose of priming it to either fight or flee. If the danger is not correctly perceived then these substances will not be released and the body will be helpless and unable to respond.

To make matters worse, aspies are much more prone to **habituation** than others. Habituation is the condition when a person stops to respond to a situation after repeated exposure. A normal person may stop responding to a sound once he or she realizes that this sound is inconsequential and presents no adverse effects. The same stands true with an image or any other external stimulus.

A normal person may even bring himself or herself to not respond to a harmful stimulus after training and special precautions have been put into place. Unfortunately, when an aspie does not comprehend the harm that may come from a stimulus, he or she may reach habituation without any provisions, training or special precautions taken to avoid being hurt.

While what we have described so far are the most dire situations, the motor and sensory perception problems may be present in simpler, everyday functions and activities that a person suffering from AS may not be able to understand.

The problems in this aspect of the syndrome were first mentioned by Asperger himself. Riding a bicycle, opening a jar, and other functions requiring even the simplest of motor dexterities are acquired after a significant delay by children suffering from AS. At the same time, aspies may move awkwardly or, as Asperger put it, **"they do not feel comfortable in their own skins."**

Their hand-to-eye coordination is poor, their motion synchronization is poor, their posture may be odd or bouncy, their handwriting may even be unreadable and they may have problems with proprioception, which is the understanding of the body's position. They are also sometimes off-balance, and if they are asked to walk in tandem gait (with the toes of the back foot touching the heel of the front foot), they may not be able to.

The next problem in reference to motor skills and sensory perception is sleep. Children with Asperger's are prone to a bad quality of sleep, frequently waking up during the night or very early in the morning. They may also have difficulty in falling asleep altogether. It is not an unusual practice for the parents of a child with AS to induce sleep by giving him or her a mild sedative or valerian.

Relevant studies have shown that 73% of AS cases experience such problems and that there may be a unique physiological reaction involved. The evidence shows that the problems in motor and sensory perception may prevent these children from reaching REM, or rapid eye movement, sleep. During a normal REM phase, the release of neurotransmitters (namely serotonin) is completely halted. The result is an almost complete paralysis of the body due to motor neuron inhibition.

This entire sequence of events is actually absent in the sleep cycles of aspies. The result is known as REM behavior disorder. People in this state actually repeat the actions of from their dreams and experience parasomnias, which are transitional stages between wakefulness and non-REM sleep. This is why most AS children are more sluggish and disoriented when they wake up.

Poor sleep is bad for any medical situation. Good quality of sleep is a well-known remedy because it allows the body to heal itself. For the children with AS, the impact is unequivocal. It prompts negative mood swings, aggravates selective attention problems and further impairs cognitive functions.

Using sedatives to remedy the sleep problems is actually a bad idea, with the exception of chamomile. Parents need to get used to the notion that their children will resist sleep at first and then they will slowly grow accustomed to these changes. So far the most effective remedies in the case of AS are physical exercise, which will tire the body and force it to seek rest, alteration of the diet and changes in the bedroom environment and the sleep routine. Parents should also be aware that when they implement these changes, the sleeping situation may get worse before it improves.

In reference to physical exercise, apart from discharging the energy of the body, there is another objective involved. For about thirty to forty-five minutes before bedtime it is recommended that there should be a period of relaxation during which all sources of stimuli, like TV, radio, computer, Xbox or PlayStation and music, should be turned off. This will decrease the arousal of the child and help him or her to sleep better. For that matter, it is even recommended that parents remove all such sources from their child's bedroom.

The recommended diet alterations for people with AS involve avoidance of any foods containing high fat and MSG (monosodium glutamate), along with large meals two to three hours before bedtime. There should also be no use alcohol, tobacco or caffeine. Instead, food rich in proteins should be consumed along with a small carbohydrate/protein snack or milk before bedtime. For the children that wake up in the middle of the night to use the bathroom and then cannot fall asleep again, fluid consumption should be restricted in the two hours before going to bed.

On the subject of changing the sleep routine, the fact the aspies follow repetitive patterns may actually come in handy, as the best course of action is to set and maintain a specific hour of going to bed and waking up each morning. This routine should include the weekends, as many parents have the bad habit of allowing their children to sleep later and wake up later on a non-school day.

When a child wakes up late, it is difficult to go to sleep at the pre-arranged time. Keep in mind that it is much easier to wake up a sleeping child than putting an active child to sleep. If a child has trouble falling asleep and does not follow repetitive patterns, the following trick can be used when the change is implemented.

The first few nights the child is allowed to sleep whenever they feel tired but his wake up time must be kept the same. At some point, he will fall asleep ten minutes after he was put to bed. When this happens, the bedtime should be moved fifteen minutes earlier. This process is to be repeated until the desired bedtime is reached.

It is important for the child that the bedroom is not associated with activity but kept strictly as a sleeping environment. Temperature should be regulated to avoid extremes and, if possible, kept at the same level constantly. Light increases are associated with corresponding decreases in the release of melatonin, which in turn, triggers the child to wake up. Thus, it is important to make arrangements so that sunlight streams in the bedroom as early in the morning as possible.

Under the same premise and of equal importance is to darken the room at nightfall. In actuality, this is a suggestion that is not limited to children with AS but can be extended to all children who have trouble falling asleep. If the child displays fear of the dark, some psychotherapy may be required. And any clocks existing inside the bedroom should be removed. Watching the time may be a stressing factor causing anxiety.

These changes will require persistence and patience, but what the parents stand to provide for their children through regulating their sleep patterns and allowing them to get good-quality sleep is priceless. Their children will be in better moods when they wake up and in general, they will be capable of sustained attention and their overall health will be improve.

Unfortunately, there may be children suffering from AS of an extreme severity for which none of the above sleep remedies may be effective. If this is the case, a sleep expert should be contacted to provide guidance and advice or provide an appropriate solution. It could also be very useful to talk to other parents of children with AS who may have relevant experience.

Some people and cultures favor a siesta. This is highly inadvisable for children with AS especially if they have difficulty falling asleep. If they sleep during the day, it will be all the more difficult to get them to sleep again when it's time to go to bed at night.

Conclusion

We have to understand that Asperger syndrome is not a disease but a syndrome or neurological condition, where a child has to face some problems in his life. But if we adopt some prevention and treatment methods as described in this book, then we can not only train our child how to live a normal life, but we can also give them a positive thought towards life. The child who lives with Asperger may look normal but his behaviour can be delusional and downright difficult to control. If we adopt the common techniques that we learn through reading of this book or other books related to Asperger syndrome, then we can teach our children how to cope with some neurological disorders of this disease. If your child is learning in his middle class or high school, then you have to give privilege to him and spend as much time as you can with him or her. Never let your child feel lonely and dumped in this condition because this may lead to severity of his or her disorders. Every child suffering from Asperger syndrome needs a different level of learning techniques and strategies to make him act normal. An individual child may show different symptoms of this syndrome depending on his age, surroundings, and his perception towards the real world. Parents need to put maximum attention to their child in this case.